ANNIE'S

MEDICAL MISADVENTURES.

Welcome to my book and to my unpleasant journey through health and the lack of it.

This is my humble account of all the mind numbing, psychologically shattering and physically shocking experiences I have suffered at the hands of medical 'experts' and their, at present, 3-dimensional way of looking at things.

The truth will out as they say and now the time has at last come where I feel ready and able to relate my stories.

Onward reader...............................

Part one - physicality

I start my stories with things that have happened to me physically (there are of course ongoing psychological ramifications attached to said physical ordeals) while in the hands of the NHS and I am taken back through my memory to my first encounter.

I am about four years old and I do not feel well especially in the stomach area and my Mother who doesn't really know what to do with me is taking me to the Doctor. This augurs in the ensuing long years of childhood where my parents don't know what to do with me and always end up taking me to the Doctor's. Doctors at this time on the planet were treated like GOD, circa approximately 1955.A lot of them were army doctors who fought to keep soldiers alive during WW2 and as it happened this particular GP, one Dr Summers, was one of them and I would say had little or no experience of diagnosing and treating little girls like me!

We approached the old grey brick Victorian house called the 'surgery' and entered through a side door into a dark corridor, we then went in to the waiting room through a door on the left. The waiting room was of a medium size with plastic seating arranged round the edge of the room and it was dark. There were numerous people in there from all walks of life. My Mother and I sat down and I felt for the first time FEAR. I didn't know what I was afraid of but the place filled me with foreboding and as I was to learn, my intuition would never let me down.

As we sat there waiting I could hear the strident tones of a woman telling a patient off for daring to walk down the corridor without first going through the waiting room procedure. The strident tones got nearer to the waiting room and then entered in the body of a middle-aged woman with red hair, piercing grey eyes and scarlet lipstick! She was wearing a white coat and held a pad of paper in one hand and a biro in the other. The piercing grey eyes scanned the waiting room and alighted on my Mother and me, she came towards us and proceeded to demand all the details of my stomach discomfort in front of all and sundry that were avidly listening. I was mortified, to me my illness was an embarrassment because it showed pathetic weakness and as an Aries(More about astrology later!) I was of the small warrior type; little did I know that my particular battles would always be with my body and the people supposed to be looking after it. After this embarrassment, it was followed by people ogling and staring at me for a few minutes and then there were others that were put through the same procedure. Then we waited and waited and my stomach churned with fear, then suddenly my name was called out by the strident voice and my Mother ushered me down the long corridor to the

Doctor's room, by this time my little heart was beating very fast and the nerves in my stomach overlaid the original problem, so much so that I couldn't tell which was which. I was small, the Doctor was tall and I could see the red veins up his nose. He and My Mother spoke to each other about my body and he boomed to me (I won't say asked... ! ?) to get up on the examining table.

This I did with the very worrying thought that maybe there wasn't anything wrong with me and I would be thought of as a TIME WASTER. I was examined, my vest pulled up and my stomach prodded and poked. As I thought, nothing was found to be out of order but just in case I was prescribed medicine and that was about it. He boomed goodbye and made a remark that was supposed to be funny which I didn't understand and my Mother and I left.

And since that day the fear has never left me when I approach a doctor.

2

What is fear one asks and the dictionary comes out, Chambers 20th Century dictionary given to me by my Dad after he bought a new one. The Meaning of fear is, according to this great tome:

" A painful emotion excited by danger"

And I think the word <u>danger</u> is the epitome of fear because certainly I instinctively felt danger when I had my first experience of doctors at such a young age. I was not aware of the exact reasons but I would learn why I felt like that as the years passed.

The orthodox medical profession offer two things to help

you get better, drugs and surgery. The first one may help but also may have deadly side effects, the second involves slicing into the body to mend or remove the affliction which may help if you have broken a bone or need a tumour or inflamed organ removing or blood vessels stitched up or unblocked. These two things address the physical body but take no account of the emotional, mental or spiritual bodies, which, dare I say, surround the physical. (See Kirlian photography.) Dare I say also that we are made up of energy, which vibrates at a certain rate, which in the 3rd dimension is quite slow and gross! Hence the sludgy treacle effect that from time to time we all feel we are trudging through down here on good old planet earth.

The other thing, which I must mention here, is the 'Tidal Flows' that operate within the physical body. As we are made up of approximately 85% water it follows that we are affected by the gravitational pull of the moon, which also governs the tides of the great oceans around the planet. The pull of the moon on our personal ocean within our physical body is as important in determining our health or lack of it as anything else such as the food and liquid we ingest and bugs such as 'flu and infections that fly around in the air we breathe. If the tide is out we become somewhat dehydrated and less able to function well, if the tide is in we may become water-logged and start to drown, metaphorically speaking. A balance in between is the ideal and at certain times of the moon month we feel better than at others.

The emotions are ruled by the element of Water and the moon month determines our emotional state, it waxes and wanes. Talking of which, everything waxes and wanes, comes and then goes including life, illness and anything else you care to think of on Gaia (Mother earth) at the moment.

But I digress. My next experience was when I accidentally swallowed a penny at the age of five. My Father had given me my pocket money in pennies, and they were the big old ones! So, in one hand the pennies, in the other a big ripe juicy plum which I was gradually munching through. At some point between eating the plum and holding the pennies, the one must have got confused with the other and I managed to put a penny in my mouth and swallowed it without realising. But, I felt this hard 'thing' in my throat and as much as I swallowed I couldn't shift it. My Mother at this point must have realised something was amiss and started asking me if I was all right, to which I could not reply properly, so she turned me upside down, thinking I must have swallowed the plum stone, in an effort to get it out, all that happened was that I was sick but the penny didn't show itself. Fortunately my Father had left the car for my Mother that afternoon and she bundled me in and drove fast up to the hospital casualty department. We sat in the waiting area and I managed to tell her that I had swallowed

a penny not a plum stone which she conveyed urgently to

the receptionist and I have never seen people move so

fast. I was immediately taken to X- Ray and then in a

matter of minutes I was up on the operating table

surrounded by at least two doctors and several nursing

staff. An instrument was put in my mouth to keep it wide

open and a huge tweezer- like instrument was put right

down my throat and eventually came back out with...'The

penny'! I just lay there looking up at the Doctor who had

probably without question just saved my life. He said 'next

time swallow a sixpence, it'll go right through!'

Everybody laughed with relief. My poor Mum, I don't know

how she has managed with me all these years as this sort

of thing has gone on and on all my life and at this time she

is ninety- four and I am sixty four!

My next experience involves a large bookcase with a glass

shutter on the front of each shelf. This particular item of furniture was kept in the then dining room of the large Victorian house we lived in, by the window.

My elder sister and I had returned from school early one afternoon, it must have been near

the end of term for us to get home at this time and we were very excited and I was goading my sister into a state of high irritability and thoroughly enjoying it as I unusually had the upper hand. Let me say at this time that my elder sister is MENSA intelligent and usually has the upper hand in most matters. However at this time I had it and was relishing the feeling of power. Pride comes before a fall and oh yes, this time it did.

My elder sister in her irritation pushed me backwards, hard, I lost my balance and fell onto one of the open bookcase glass shutters and went through it. The glass shattered and my Mum came running in from the kitchen.

I was pulled out of the shards of glass and I stood up, my Mum asked if I was ok. I felt ok but when we looked down at the side of my school dress there was a big hole in it, there was also a big hole in my knickers and under neath those there was a big hole in me with a large piece of glass sticking out of it. In fact there were two holes in me, one, a jagged crooked hole and the other, a long straight hole and there was blood, lots of it.

My older sister just looked and I don't know how she felt, but it was my fault for goading her and I had got myself into a situation that was not going to be enjoyable.

My Mother ran out of the house and over the road to where the aforementioned tall, red veined nose GP lived, he came over, as he happened to be in at the time, and came into the house and again towered over me and looked at my wounds, he boomed that they were deep and I would need to go to the hospital. At this point the FEAR set in and the shock, I suspect, and I started crying. So once more it was down to my Mum. She hadn't got the car that afternoon and had to run next door to ask if she could borrow the next door neighbour's Heinkel called Hetty. This was a bubble car and those with good memories will recall these very small noisy German cars! However that afternoon my Mum would have to learn very quickly how to drive this weird car. We got in through the door on the front of the car sat down and then closed it; I had a large wad of cotton wool attached to my derrière. Mum had to find the gears and back it out of the driveway. Mum had driven lorries in the war so she probably was ok! We buzzed our way to the hospital and again entered the waiting area in casualty.

I was seen quickly and again ushered onto a treatment table and was greeted by a female doctor. She had a good look at the holes in my left buttock and said that the straight slash would be easy to stitch but the crooked one would be harder. She prepared the area, swabbed it down with alcohol to clean it and dabbed it with lint and then advanced towards me with a large curved needle threaded with catgut. I lay on the table, gaunt and stiff with fear with my Mum standing behind me and holding my shoulders. The needle went in-ouch- and then came out the other side-ouch and the catgut was tied.

That was stitch number one. In those days they didn't give you a shot of anaesthetic to numb the area - why???.

Number two stitch went in - urrrrr - and came out - urrrrr.

Number three stitch went in- aahhh- and came out- aaahhh.

By this time I had had enough and said as much. I was told that I was to have five more stitches in the crooked hole, the straight hole was done. Quite frankly I don't know how I got through those five stitches and probably wouldn't have done without my Mum holding on to me. The pain was excruciating and I screamed my way through the rest of the experience. Why couldn't they have given me a local anaesthetic......!? Perhaps they actually enjoyed inflicting pain onto people and little girls; that was a distinct possibility.

Afterwards we drove back in Hetty Heinkel, deposited her in her own driveway and got home. I was off school for a week after that episode and had to be careful of the stitches. They came out, when they did, with much more ease than they had gone in !

So, the Penny and the Glass shutter, two supposed accidents but as I know now there are no accidents really just very fast reasons for things happening and mostly down to human error. Lack of concentration the first and a sense of power and pride the next, both down to me.

3

This is where things start to get tricky and serious for me.
When I was seven (1958)we went on holiday to Lyme Regis
in Dorset. I just loved it there; I would spend hours sitting
at the end of the 'Cobb' (harbour wall) with my feet
dangling over the edge watching the sea below crashing
onto the rocks and when the tide was out watching people
climbing on those rocks. I also watched the boats coming
and going from the harbour, fishing boats, lobster boats,
yachts, canoes, Royal Navy patrol boats and Boat trip
boats!

Sometimes I would climb on the rocks with my older sister
but usually I was on my own.
That last year there would be my last normal year mentally

for a very long time. As I walked for the last time on the Cobb back to my parents on the beach I felt something bad was coming, didn't know what it was but I felt unease.

The year after(1959) we went on holiday to Jersey in the Channel Islands. It was very exciting because we were going by large ferry from Weymouth at night. We travelled to Weymouth by car, which was then loaded onto the ferry by a crane. We had a late meal in a cafeteria and my Mum tried to get me to swallow a travel sickness pill, I just couldn't get it down and in the end spat it out when she wasn't looking!

We then embarked upon our journey making our way onto the ferry. My Dad had booked us reclining seats so we could sleep. The ferry set off and we left England's shores. I slept fitfully during that night, mainly due to excitement and also a storm that had kicked up about halfway across the English Channel. The ferry rocked back and forth and I became wide awake so much so that I went for a walk and ventured nearly onto the deck, but the spray from the sea prevented me from trying it, also the thought of being washed overboard! We arrived at St Helier at the beginning of the next day, the main town on Jersey where we docked and got off the ferry. We watched as the car was unloaded by another crane and then we started our holiday. We stayed in a downstairs holiday flat near St Ouen's Bay. We went to the beach quite often and also travelled round the island to have a look at places of note, one of which was the old German Underground Hospital. The tunnels and the history of the place fascinated me. This, I think, but can't quite remember, was the last day of feeling ok. The next day we went to a different beach and as I sat there with my family I knew something was wrong with me because my perception of the world had changed from being free, normal and sharp to being distorted and limited, also my head felt odd.

How do you tell your parents that your mind and your head don't feel right? I don't know and I certainly did not know at the age of eight because I didn't understand what had happened to me, all I knew was that I didn't feel right anymore in my head, I couldn't think clearly and the world had become a dull and distorted grey place for me. This huge change happened overnight, one day I was fine the next I most certainly was not. Did my parents notice that I was not myself during the rest of that holiday, probably but they didn't mention it to me. We spent the last night of the holiday in St Helier and returned to England the next day on the ferry.

4

I was not coping at school, I couldn't concentrate and I was finding it harder to do things like mental arithmetic. Another thing that I noticed was how I felt after we had been for swimming lessons. We had to walk to the Swimming Baths uphill and back again. I found that I was not able to keep up with my peers when we were swimming and when we got back to school I seemed to always have a gurgling indigestion and usually ended up lying flat on my back on the grass during break time to try and get rid of it. Whether it was the chlorine in the pool or whether the exertion of the swimming and walking that did it I don't know but it was very difficult for me as I was trying to hide from the people around me that I was struggling with my health. In those days, the early 1960's, people's ideas of health or lack of it were very weird. Also my dread of the doctors was quite pronounced now. I was frightened as well because I didn't know what the problem was with me and couldn't seem to talk to anyone about it. I was kept down the following year in the Middle School because my grades had fallen, thus mirroring my difficulty in keeping up with everyone else. I think my parents by this time were beginning to realise that I was struggling. I was taken to the red veined doctor who examined me and said I was highly strung and gave me some pills to calm me down. I was fed these pills each day, which became a nightmare because I couldn't swallow them. I think my Mum crunched them up in the end with some jam and I was forced to swallow them like that.

I have to say that it is difficult for me to write all this down as it is bringing back very difficult memories, some of which I had forgotten until now. I don't know if the pills helped or not but I continued to get the bus to School in Northampton at 8.00 am and do a full day's studying and catch the 4.30pm bus back and get home at 5.30pm in Kettering – a long day. On top of that I had to do my homework after supper. It was all getting too much for me and I was taken back to the doctor who gave me some brown iron tablets as he thought I was anaemic. No further investigations were done at this time. My mental state was deteriorating even more and there would be big 'emotional outbursts'.

I knew there was something wrong with me but I didn't know what it was and neither did the red veined doctor and he didn't seem moved to find out either. How ill do you have to get before these people will take intelligent considered action...?! My work at school deteriorated even further and I was now in the Main school (Senior). I couldn't bear the thought of going to school anymore on the bus because I felt travel sick and also I was not managing to do my homework and I had to make up excuses for not doing it to my teachers. My Father and I had outrageous arguments about me going to school and I was dragged kicking and screaming to the car to get me there because I had missed the bus. There was one occasion when he thrashed me on my backside, in those days that's what parents did to offending children, at least in my family that's what happened. I have to say that my younger sister was witness to all this and also had to come to the school with us in the car sometimes. My older sister must have been witness to all of this as well although I would think she kept pretty much out of it, she always did and still does!

What, you may ask, was the GP doing about all this, sweet FA, that is what. Meanwhile things got worse, I was so tired all the time, tired in my body, tired in my mind, tired in my spirit and I was only eleven (1962). I felt about 90.

The Headmistress meanwhile was taking note of the number of times I was in the Medical Room and came in to see me in there quite a few times. One of the worst times was when I started vomiting and having diarrhoea at the same time and the school sent me home on the bus where I was also sick and had diarrhoea all at the same time. Fortunately the bus conductor was female and did her best to comfort me and even walked me home at the end of the journey, my pants were full and it was hard to walk. My mum was appalled at the state of me and gave me a bath and put me to bed and stayed with me until my dad came home .She was very angry at the School for sending me home on my own on a bus in my quite dreadful condition, they hadn't explained the severity of my symptoms to her or they had underestimated them. I had a week off School, thank god. I could at last rest my poor weary body, my sick mind and sleep.

5

The nightmare continued, I became quite clumsy and would knock my glass of water over at the dinner table often. The headmistress summoned my parents to talk to them about me. Obviously I was not coping at school and also I was clearly not well, what were they going to do about it. She could no longer accommodate me in her school. My parents asked her for advice on where I should go to school, as I had to be educated by law. Places were named and suggestions given.

Meanwhile the red veined GP had arranged an appointment for me to see the child psychiatrist, he obviously thought it was all in my mind, at the local NHS Clinic. I didn't want to go, I had had enough of being looked at, poked and prodded by the medical profession. My parents dragged me literally to the appointment where I was seen by a nurse and then I was tested for my IQ during which I cried because I couldn't do some of the things that involved shapes and holes and puzzles of where to put the pieces together.

Then I was ushered into another room and interviewed by the child psychiatrist. He was of medium build, dressed in a black suit and white shirt and dark tie. He wore glasses and peered at me for a while. What he made of me I don't know, I told him that I just didn't want to leave my Mum, I felt as if I was in an incredibly difficult examination in which there were no accurate answers, but the outcome produced several things, one was that I should be able to manage to go to school locally at the secondary modern and also the idea was put forward that maybe my home life didn't suit me. So now my family were the fault. In short it was probably all in my mind and a few adjustments should make me feel better.

My poor parents had to take on this opinion and it must have hit them hard, again in those days doctors were God and you obeyed.

Meanwhile I still felt ill! The psychiatrist I saw in November 1962 and things moved on to find me alternative schooling. The first time I was aware of this was a real shock because no one had mentioned anything to me. I came down the stairs one evening from my bedroom and noticed a pile of A4 brown envelopes on the hall chair. I was drawn to them and had a quick furtive peek inside them, my heart sank as I realised I was looking at boarding school prospectuses. There were about five or six in all. I was totally shocked and very upset that my parents were considering the possibility that I should be sent away from home to boarding school. They had obviously taken on the opinion of the psychiatrist that my home life didn't suit me. I marched into the sitting room where my family were talking and confronted them with the envelopes and screamed at them for even considering sending me away. My Father said "Now Anne, that's enough" in a stern voice, my Mum didn't say anything. I felt devastated that they would send me away. I felt that they didn't love me anymore and they just wanted to be rid of me because I had become a hindrance because I was unwell and my mental state was precarious. The state of my mind was to say the least very odd and the bad emotional outbursts continued. I became very depressed and felt isolated from my family. The doctors had given up on me and now my family had.

That's how it was for me.

6

The month was February, the year 1963. The weather was extremely cold and there were icicles on the trees. We drove carefully towards Warwickshire, as the roads were very slippery. My parents were taking me for an interview at a Boarding School the other side of Warwick on the road between Warwick and Solihull, Birmingham.
The school was called Wroxall Abbey School.

We turned off the road and through the main school gates and drove down a very long straight drive.

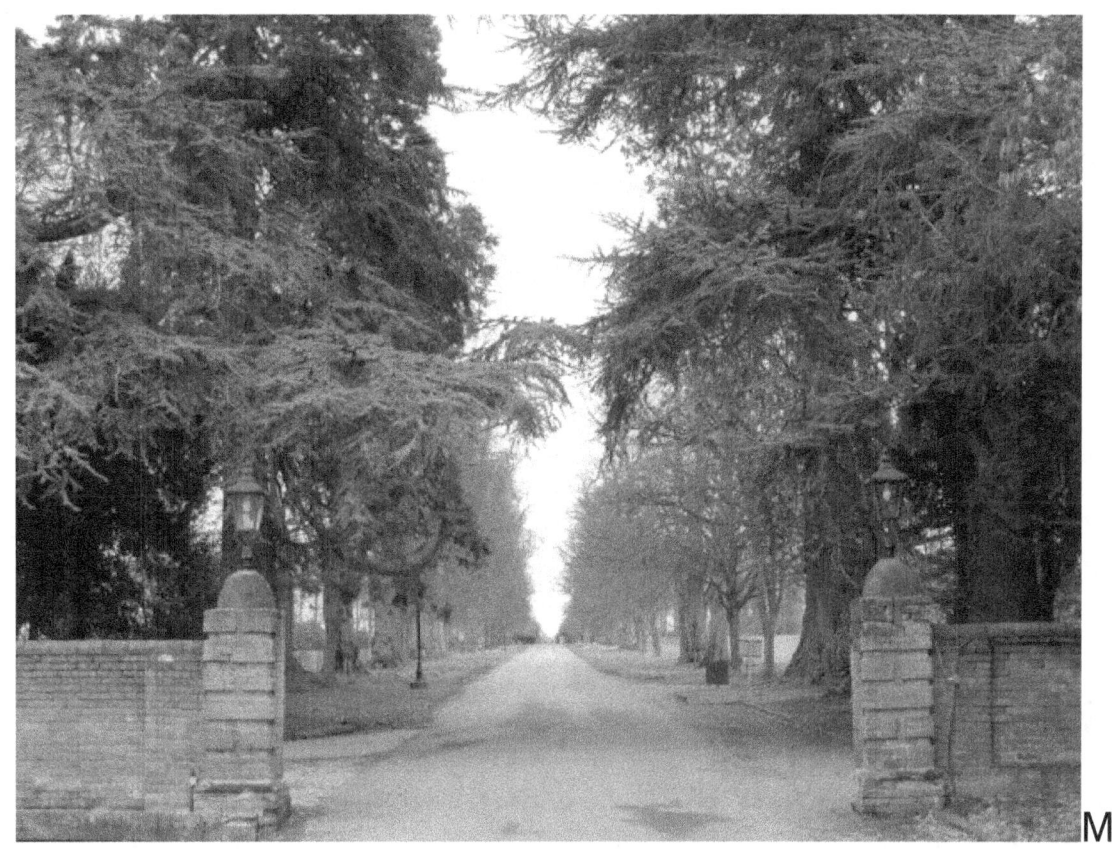

M

y Mum was trying to encourage me by pointing out the frozen lake and the sports field. Everywhere was white with frost and snow. I felt ill and very depressed and very scared. My Dad drove the car to the front door of a huge imposing Mansion.

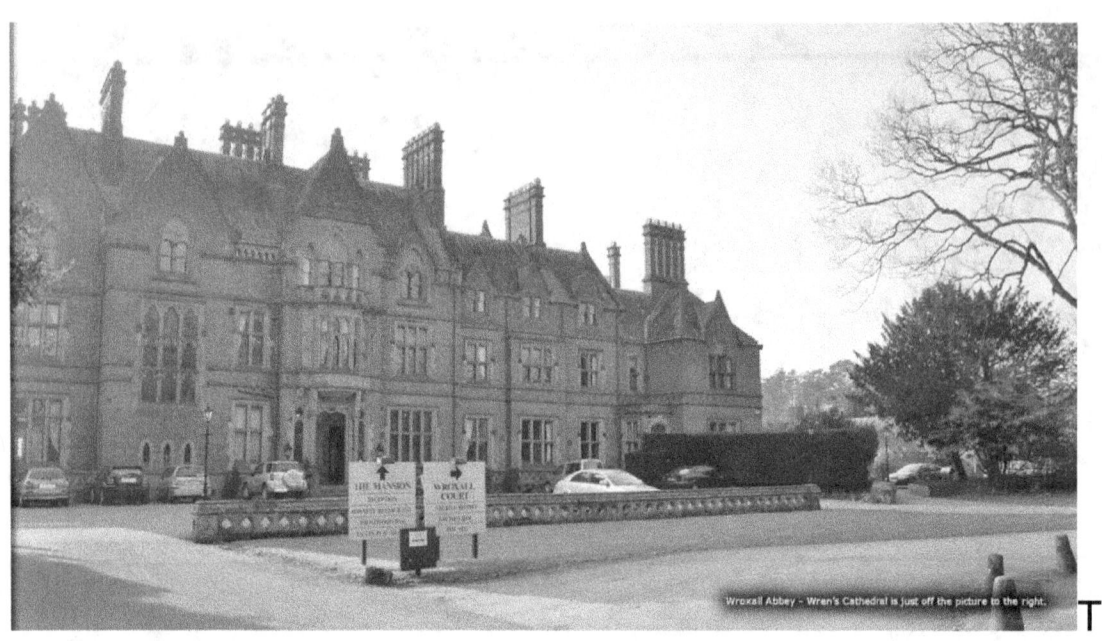

Wroxall Abbey - Wren's Cathedral is just off the picture to the right.

This was it then, the nightmare was growing. I was ushered in with my parents by the headmistress and up a huge oaken staircase. We sat in her study while they talked about me and then I was taken by her to a small room where I was tested for Maths and English and my reading abilities. The maths was crap and the English was fine and lo and behold – I could read! She said my reading was good, I think she was surprised.

I think we looked around the place but my memory of that is gone.

We left and drove home, but I have very little memory of that too.

The school had accepted me and there was a flurry of activity as my parents started to get all the things I would need. Mum and I had a trip up to Peter Jones the department store in Sloane Square, London to buy all the uniform.

I don't remember much of this time except that I didn't feel well and I had the prospect looming of being away from my family. I felt very alone. No one seemed to care about me and I think they would be relieved when I was no longer at home. It would mean their lives could get back to normal and they wouldn't have to worry about me anymore.

7

I entered Wroxall Abbey School in April 1963 aged twelve.

Thin, homesick and in the wrong uniform! Everyone else was wearing the smart blue suits but my Mother had put me into a pleated navy skirt and navy cardigan with a white shirt and tie. I felt mortified as I stood out as a new girl and in odd clothes. At that age it is important that you fit in and that means the right clothes! My parents came to bid me goodbye after talking to the headmistress and I felt a wave of homesickness wash over me, (don't leave me, Mum). They went and I unpacked my trunk. I was put in a bedroom with five other girls and that included the head of bedroom, a fifth year girl called Jackie Dare. She was quite attentive towards me and tried to cheer me up as I cried myself to sleep for the first week of my first term there. I was introduced to the concept of Dame Alice, a ghost that walked round the school and a baby's head rolling down the corridors.

I became quite alarmed at this, but the other girls laughed behind my back as they built the story up into something large in my head.

I sort of settled into the school or tried to. I didn't make any special friends that term and felt lonely. On days out with my Mum and Dad I would tear off the ankle socks, which made me feel like a two year old and put on stockings. At half term the time went so fast when I was at home and I couldn't stop thinking that I would have to go back to the school in four days time and the homesickness would start again. I got through that first term, my report was inconsequential and just said that I could do better. I had good marks for piano, English, art and dance, everything else was a struggle.

I was so glad to be home for the school holidays, six weeks - home, phew!
It went by quickly, I read a lot and didn't do much, and then it was September and time to return to Wroxall. I was

still over thin and found eating a chore. In my mind I had retreated into a dark compartment where I was untouchable and protected from the people out there that didn't know what was wrong with me and played with their diagnoses. My body might be theirs to play with but my mind (even though it wasn't right) and spirit were my own. Back to school I went. Three weeks into the term quite a few of us fell ill with a gastric bug and we had to stay in bed. Time went on and the others got better.

Me? I just stayed the same and my temperature wouldn't go down. After 2 weeks like this I was moved into the school sanatorium, I was the only one in there. I lost about two and a half stone very quickly over the next ten days and found it impossible to eat much although the school matron tried to get me to eat more. I would hide some of the food in my bag so she wouldn't get at me about it, Mum had to fumigate the bag later on. During this time my parents visited me. They sat far away from me and ignored my crying pleas to go home. They said it was up to the school. (So now the school was God).

I think at this time the headmistress was beginning to get quite worried about me and she arranged for two medical specialists to come in and examine me. I was stripped of my bedclothes and my nightdress by the matron and lay naked on the sanatorium bed. The matron, headmistress and the two male doctors peered down at my emaciated naked body and the doctors started to poke and prod me all over including my groin and under my arms. I felt mortified and very scared and ill. The doctors left with the headmistress and the matron helped me to get my nightdress on and then covered me with the bedclothes, I remember the smell of the fusty blankets. I was left on my own to ponder the possible outcome of this visit.

The next day a portable X-Ray machine was brought in

with a radiographer and pictures were taken of my body and a while after that, maybe a day or two, I was visited by one of the specialists that had examined me. He came in on his own and sat close to me. He explained to me that 'shadows' had been found on my lungs and that they needed to find out what they were exactly and for that I would need to go into hospital. I was given the choice of either Warwick General Hospital or going home to Kettering General Hospital. I chose home. My parents came to take me back to Kettering and I was bundled into a red blanket and carried down the main Oak staircase. My Class came to say goodbye to me and then I was put in the back of the car. My parents were very worried and were also very stressed as the onus of responsibility for me had been placed squarely back on their shoulders. They were to take me straight to the hospital with no side visits to home although I was upset because I was hoping to see my rabbit and cuddle her soft furry body before being taken to the hospital but my Father was adamant, straight to the hospital.

8

The next stage of my young life had begun–<u>Hospitals.</u> My dad and I entered the main door to Kettering General Hospital. Upon enquiry, they didn't seem to know who I was or have any information about me. One wonders if any of them communicated with each other. My dad was getting more and more stressed and angry and I had to cope with him as well as the fact that I thought I was going to faint. Eventually I was taken to a women's medical ward and put in a bed about halfway down the long corridor like room. There was a line of beds down each side of the ward. The curtains were drawn around the bed next to me where a poor woman was having a lumbar puncture. The crying and moaning at the pain of it coming from her scared me and again I became gaunt and stiff as I lay there. I think my

Dad must have gone and I can't remember anything about my Mum on that day.

I was moved to a small side ward later that evening as I was clearly too young to be in the main ward and too old to be in the children's ward. Thus began the observation of my body, all urine and faeces were to be kept and examined. The whole of my body was X-rayed, and every three days I was required to swallow a naso-gastric tube from which they would suck out the contents of my stomach which would then be analysed. This particular procedure was appalling and would be carried out at about 5.00am as night turned into day. I managed the first time, just about, but the second and third times I just couldn't tolerate it, they forced it down the second time and the third I screamed at them and demanded that a doctor should do it. A doctor did come to see me and decided that it was not required any more; I presume they had enough evidence from the previous two excursions into my stomach contents

to be able to come to some prognosis. Every so often they

would want to take a sputum test which would require me

to let them place a long thin glass tube down the back of

my throat and I would have to cough onto the piece of lint

that was at the end of the glass tube on a wire. I didn't

have a productive cough at the time and I don't know if

they got a good enough sample with which to make a

diagnosis.

I was in the general hospital for over two weeks and they

still hadn't come to a diagnosis. My Father was furious

enough to call the child specialist at the local golf club on a

Sunday and interrupt his game and demand that he come

up with an answer. I was told this years later.

He did. On the Tuesday after the golf club incident a

Specialist, One Dr Fisher, on his own, who proceeded to

tell me that I had tuberculosis in both lungs, visited me. The disease had started on the outside of my lungs and burrowed its way towards the inside of my lungs since the initial infection. I was told later in my life that they reckoned I had had it for nearly two years before it was discovered. (What, you may wonder, was the GP playing at? I have wondered that many times over the years, he should have been struck off!)

Consumption! – This explained to me why I had been feeling so bad all this time; I was being consumed little by little. It did not however totally explain my mental state, which had deteriorated into full-blown depression as well as distortion. Obviously the TB itself did not help my state of mind, but there was another undetected reason for my difficult mental state, which would remain so for many years to come.

I was also told that I would have to go to another hospital to be looked after while I had tuberculosis. This was a specialist chest hospital in a town called Rushden, twelve miles away; they said I would be there a month so as not to frighten me further, in fact I was there for seven and a half months.

The next day came and I was transported to the chest hospital in an ambulance with my Mother to keep me company. We arrived and I was taken to a small single room with large French windows looking out onto a green lawn; the trees were losing their leaves. I sat on the edge of the bed feeling very frightened because the thought of being on my own freaked me out. I conveyed this to my Mum and burst into tears. My Mum was so worried about me, I think she would have done anything to help me get used to this new place and had a word with the Sister and asked if I could be with other people. The Sister, by some miracle, understood and had me moved to quite a large ward in a different building. I was the youngest person there and the nearest in age was a young woman of sixteen, from the town of Corby, also with tuberculosis and also very pregnant!

For three weeks I was not allowed out of bed. I lay there in bed, resting and listening to the conversations of the women around me, I remember one Lady who had an enormous scar down her back and round to her front. She told me that she had had her lung removed because the tuberculosis had eaten all the way through it and that there was nothing else they could do. Most of us were on medication, strong drugs that consisted of a streptomycin injection every morning in the derriere! Another drug, which looked like pink birdseed in small packets, was given to us everyday. It tasted and smelled absolutely foul and I found it impossible to get it down my throat, everything in me repelled it and I would gag violently.

Nobody checked if I was taking it and I hid the packets in the locker next to my bed! Of course they were found eventually and the specialist was told. He was a lovely gentle Scottish man called Dr Gerard who was acquainted with my Father through Rotary and I was put on some new medicine called Pasinah D. This was a powder in strawberry or lime flavour, which had to be dissolved in a glass of water. I chose strawberry, it tasted almost as abominable as the birdseed but at least it didn't get stuck in my throat. I could manage this. Every so often we would line up in the corridor to be weighed and then the specialist would see us, this started for me about a month after I was admitted to the hospital. I weighed about four and a half stone to begin with, which was about three stone below the normal weight for my height. I was then taken in to see the specialist who talked to me and then I had to stand behind a moving picture x-ray machine so that he could see how my lungs were when I was breathing in and out. Blood was taken occasionally and my throat was examined and my teeth. The drugs could affect the way my teeth were growing and leave brown marks on them as well. My mouth was overcrowded with teeth both bottom and top and I had been told by my own dentist that I would have to have four teeth out to make room for the others; this was before the TB event happened. When I saw the dentist in hospital he was appalled at the overcrowding but I was able to convince him that my own dentist was dealing with the matter. The thought of having four teeth out at the same time as trying to fight TB was horrendous to me. I just didn't have the strength to go through that ordeal on any level physical, emotional, mental or spiritual. Fortunately my parents were consulted and reassured the hospital that things were in hand on the matter of teeth!

I also contracted tonsillitis and was terrified that I would have to have my tonsils removed, I cried while my specialist inspected them to make sure there was no TB lurking in them, again fortunately for me there was none, at least, none that they could see and I was spared surgery at that time.

My first day out of bed was on the 22 November 1963 .I was allowed to go into the common room with a blanket round me and watch some television. It was just after 4pm and there was a news flash. John F Kennedy the American President had been shot in the head in Dallas Texas. We all just sat there stunned at the news. I was quite interested in politics and had had a good feeling about Kennedy all the time he was President. This was quite awful and I felt sick in the pit of my stomach. I think everyone else did too, we were in shock. The whole world was in shock.

Time travelled on and Christmas got near, I was told that I

would be allowed home for two days over Christmas. I was glad but when the time came for me to be at home I felt pretty weak and ill and I felt sorry for my family who had to tip toe round me and look after me, especially my Mum. I was taken back to the hospital and I settled back into the routine of injections, drugs, x- rays, being poked and prodded and looked at by the specialist, weighed, watered and fed, bit like a prize Cow at a show! Every so often I would have to go through the barbaric ordeal of having to cough onto the piece of lint, which was stuck down my throat via the thin glass tube. They never managed to get any sputum worth looking at, as the TB was more on the outside of my lungs.

My weight gradually started to improve and I felt a bit more like walking around. My Dad had arranged for a Vicar called Ambrose to come in and see me and try to teach me some English and Maths as my brain still had to be nourished with numbers and words! Mostly he and I spent the time talking about philosophical matters and rarely did any anything else. This was good. My Mum brought my music case in with all the music I had been learning at School plus some other stuff like Snow White and the Seven Dwarfs and Hans Christian Andersen songs from the film about him such as 'Inch worm' and I was allowed to walk down to another building in my dressing gown with a large room with a sort of stage in it with a grand piano on the stage and I played listlessly as I felt very low in energy and also low in spirit. Something that used to give me pleasure no longer seemed to as the depression of consumption and the other thing affecting my mind, yet to be diagnosed, often took over.

In the February I started my periods, a lady patient from one of the other wards helped me to find sanitary pads and reassured me that I was doing fine. I remember her face clearly and her kindness. The period lasted for seven days and was heavy with quite severe tummy pains .I just thought here is something else I have to deal with. I rarely had any visitors except for my parents; my friends and their parents were too scared to come or get involved in case they caught the disease. My Mum came to see me everyday and my Dad came often. My Dad bought my Mum a black Ford Anglia so that she could drive over and see me. She drove through all kinds of weather, snow, ice, rain and bad fog without a car heater, how she did it I don't know but she must have loved me a lot to do that for me. I appreciated it I really did and have thanked her many times over the years. There was only one day when she didn't come to see me in all the seven months I was in the hospital. My Sister's never came.

March came and quite a few of us were getting better, my weight had gone up to over 6 stone and my appetite was improving. We still got weighed and still got injected by a lovely staff nurse who knew just how to do it without causing any bruising, but every Wednesday the Sister would do the injections and every Thursday we would all have large purple bruises on our derrieres! That woman just did not know how to inject...

The Vicar came and went and everything else came and went. By the end of the month I was deemed fit enough by the Scottish specialist to leave hospital, which I did. My colour had come back into my cheeks and I was quite bouncy.

My parents told me that I would be going back to Wroxall for the summer term. I felt ok'ish about this and quite excited to see my class mates, after all, the last time they had seen me was way back in October looking thin and gaunt.

I spent the Easter holidays enjoying being at home. My

older sister was moody and into smoking and boys. My Younger Sister was small and cute.

9

After all this, a period of respite from illness came to me. I was glad and although I would have to take Pasinah D for another four years I was able to start to enjoy my life more. Life at school improved and I made one or two close friends whom I could have a good laugh with. I wasn't allowed to do sport and had to 'walk the drive'

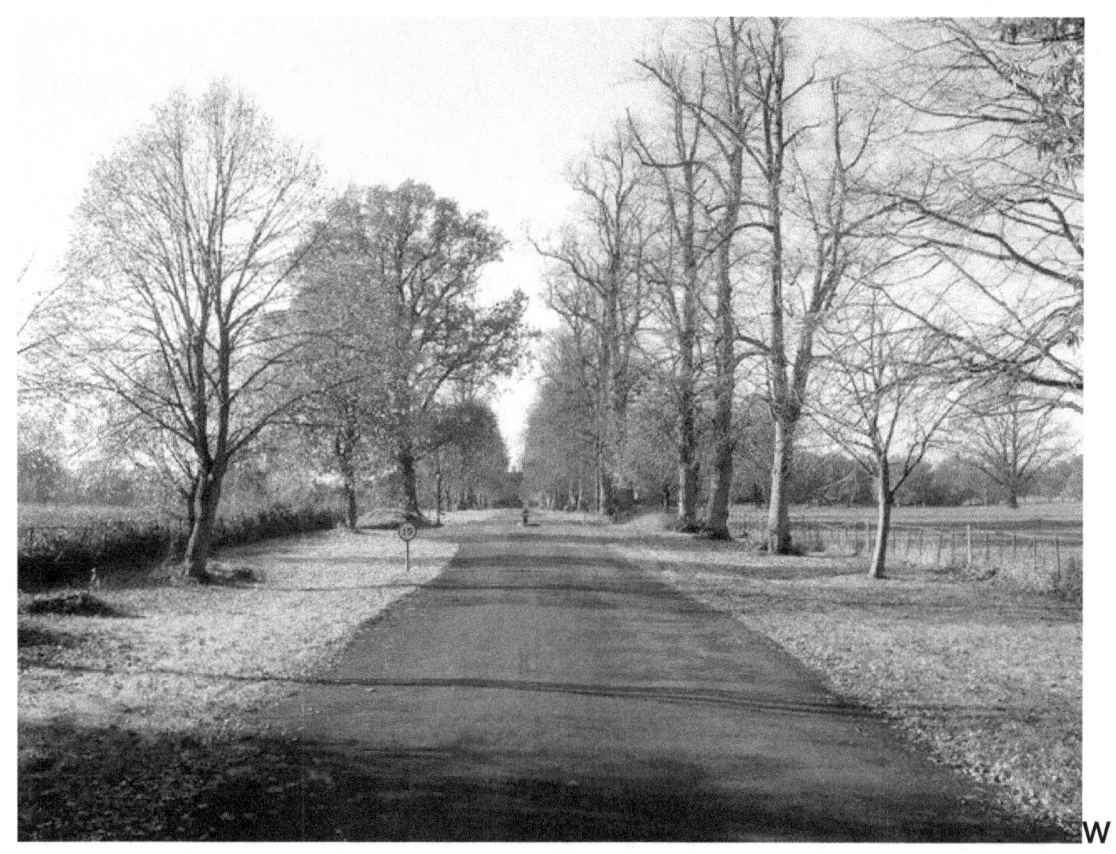W

hile everyone else played tennis or swam in the new pool. I still suffered from homesickness at the beginning of school terms but I would get over it and pour myself into whatever was going on. I learned that during my time in hospital everyone had had to have a TB test and X-Rays and that the local milk had also had to be tested in case it carried the infection. Nothing was found but people were disgruntled about it and one Irish girl had refused the TB test. As I had been ill for a long time I doubted that it had come from anything at the school.

I discovered that I was good at acting and gained a coveted place in the Drama Club when I was in the third year. I played the 'Judge' in ' Toad of Toad Hall' and also had a part in a musical called 'School and Crossbones.' I was given the main part of the boy in 'The Boy and The Bishop' much to my surprise in the fourth year and gained much commendation from the audience over my representation of the mute boy that learned to speak.

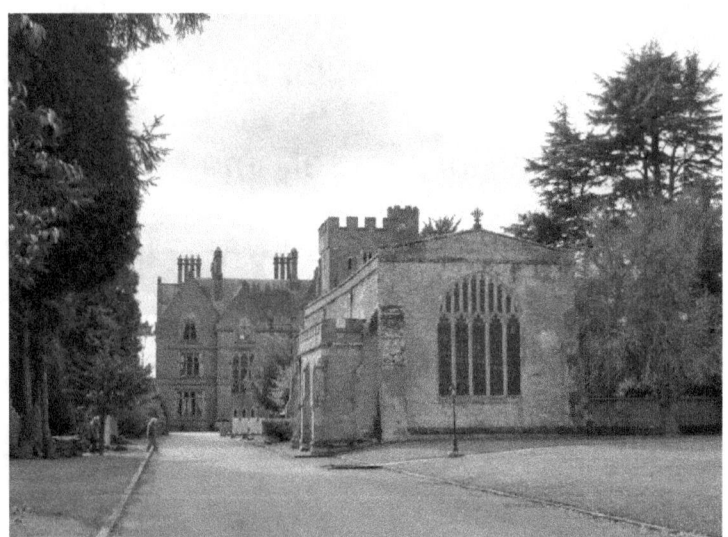

I was also good at dancing and learned how to do Irish Dancing, which we displayed at one of the Speech Days.

I enjoyed art and also writing stories. I played the Piano and passed Grade 4 and then went on to pass Grade 5. In my last year there we had GCSE exams coming up and we all had to work hard. I passed all my mock exams. In the last Term at Wroxall I ran into trouble with my peers, I had noticed that every term somebody would be picked on, usually someone that was considered weak or 'different'. Unfortunately after four and a half years at this place it was my turn to suffer at the hands of others in my class. I was sent to 'Coventry' meaning that no one would talk to me at all. I began to feel isolated and even my best friend was influenced by the others and drifted over to their side of the coin.

I wrote home and told my parents about the treatment I was getting. I couldn't focus on my work and revision and at prep times in the evenings I would immerse myself in a story that I was writing and pass it round for people to read rather than revise.

The exams came and I was the only one taking Music at O level and sat in a small room at the desk with the French teacher invidulating. Music was the only O level I passed at that School.

I had had enough and my parents could see that my time there was over and let me leave.

I returned home for the summer holidays and we went to Northern Spain, a place called Zarouz and camped in a campsite on top of a large hill overlooking the bay. My best friend from school had agreed to come with us as she had left school as well and when asked about the way the others had treated me in that last term dismissed it all as very stupid but wouldn't divulge the real reason and I am still as much in the dark now as I was then but I was perceived as weak and that was enough.

We met two gorgeous Spanish boys and went out with them quite often or they would come to the beach and swim with us, quite often we would go far beyond the waves into deep water and I would feel somewhat scared and definitely out of my depth! Mine was called Jesus; I can't remember what hers was called! We would go down to the town in the evenings and meet up with them and usually end the evenings in the sand dunes having a good snog!

Then one day they didn't show up and we learned that they had gone to Pamplona for the Bull racing festival. All the young local men went to try their hand at defeating the great bulls. We were sad because we knew that we would be going back to England and wouldn't see them again. I will always remember Jesus.

Home then and a new term at the local Technical College. I

had to do all my retakes and I had to have all the stuff

crammed into my noodle!

This was very different to Boarding School and there were

boys. I went out with quite a few over the next year and a

half and had some fun. I had finished taking Pasinah D but

had to go each year for a check up at the hospital and an

X -Ray. It eventually got to every five years and now I

haven't had an X-ray for that in years.

Am I better from it? I am, but the trauma has never left me

and the physical weakness is still with me at the age of 64

because of the scarring on my lungs.

I managed to pass the rest of my O levels and left the

'Tech'. I got a job at the local library helped by my dad

who knew the chief librarian and I earned seven pounds a

week! I worked long hours sometimes till 8 pm and also looked after the music library, which was quiet most of the time.

Sometimes I had to work in the reference library, which was quite demanding, as the phone would ring a lot and people wanted to know all sorts of things, which I would have to go and look up. Some late evenings I would work on the Main Desk and interact with all the people bringing their books back and taking new ones out. I enjoyed stamping the books and searching for the library cards. I avoided the main Telephone Switch Board as much as I could .I was shy at talking to people and also wasn't quite sure how to put someone through to someone else!

When I was seventeen I met for the first time the brother of a friend of mine around Christmas time, I certainly didn't know the huge part this brother was going to play in my life. After Christmas in the January and February I tried for

Drama School in London and Birmingham and failed to get in. My Local authority was not keen on giving grants for the Arts and wouldn't say that I would definitely get one to go to the Schools I auditioned with. I was heartbroken that I hadn't made it because of that and sank into a depression. That summer in 1969 I left my job at the library as my tonsils were playing up and My Mum had taken me to a throat specialist who said they would have to come out. I had an infection in them about once a month and even had a quinsy during one attack. I also found out I was allergic to penicillin as I was covered in a rash one morning after taking it. After the respite from illness it seemed that my body was beginning to take over again. I went privately at the General hospital and had my own room. There was another young woman in the room next door and we talked a lot the evening before the operation. The Sister chased me back to bed at about 10 pm.

The next day I was wheeled down the corridor to the

Operating Theatre, I was second on the list. We entered the anaesthetic room and the surgeon came to see me and tried to reassure me. I was injected in a vein in my right hand, I felt the stuff going up my arm and into my head, it was very unpleasant and then I suppose, nothing, until I came round back in my bed. My tongue felt huge and very dry and I could hardly swallow. I was allowed a small drink of water. It took two days for my tongue to feel the right size. I came out of the anaesthetic slowly and began to feel the pain in my throat where the tonsils had been removed. I had a look in the mirror and saw the cauterisation that had been done to stop any bleeding where my tonsils had been. I was given aspirin in the form of chewing gum, which kept a constant supply of painkiller going down my throat. I began to recover but had a relapse after some friends who talked and talked and expected me to talk and talk back visited me! My throat ached for two days after that.

My Tonsils were sent to the Pathology Lab to be checked for TB, fortunately they were found to be clear of it.

I was in the hospital for about six days and then went home, I felt tired all the time and had to rest a lot. It took about six weeks to recover. By this time it was August and I had arranged with my boyfriend, the brother aforementioned of my friend to go on holiday to North Wales. We set off and stayed in really nice hotels to begin with and then the money started to run out and we ended the holiday in bed and breakfasts that had seen better days.

During that holiday I asked him to get married to me, I had failed at the drama schools and felt that the only option open to me was to get married. He seemed to have doubts but wouldn't talk to me about them, if I had had my wits about me I would have realised that he really didn't want to but the mental problems that I still had were in the way. We went to Manchester and bought an engagement ring, second hand, a ruby surrounded by diamonds. We also bought the wedding ring. I sent a postcard to my parents saying that we were engaged. I was only eighteen and he was twenty-one. I must have been mad and so must he but we went with it and he even got christened. We were married at the beginning of December 1969 in a small village church and then had the reception at a local hotel in our hometown. There were about fifty guests. They waved goodbye to us as we set off in the car on our life journey together. Somebody had blown the tyres up too high and put a kipper in the radiator! You can imagine the stench. We had a short honeymoon in the Cotswolds and I woke up the day after the wedding wondering if I had done the right thing and I am sure he did. Neither of us said anything about that and I suppose we just got on with it.

We enjoyed our first couple of weeks together in our new

life leading up to Christmas and I tried to cook. I hadn't got a clue how to boil potatoes or an egg or anything but I would go to the supermarket and buy Vesta curries, anything from beef through to prawns. We loved those curries, they were hot and spicy. While my husband was at work I would listen to records, especially Simon and Garfunkel, I would sing 'Bridge over troubled water' again and again! I had time on my hands and didn't know anyone. I was bored during the days and started eating to pass the time, in those days there was no daytime TV.

Just before Christmas we went to my husband's company Christmas office party. When we got there I was immediately handed a huge glass of Martini and gin and several more during the course of the evening. I don't really remember the party but I remember driving home in the MGA sports car and I was drunk.

When we got in I was sick and the room was spinning. I lay on the bed and then he was on top of me having his husbandly way and forgetting or deliberately not using a condom. Nine months later, to the day, I gave birth to our Son.

I started a new job after that Christmas working in the National Westminster Bank in Stockport. I had to get up at six in the morning and get the bus from outside the bed-sit about seven which took me to the main road from Manchester through to Stockport, get on another bus and then get off that one and walk to the bank. I would get there about 8.15 am and join the other girls working there in the staff room. We would have a coffee and then get to work. I was put on a desk where I would have to go through piles of cheques and then docket them. One of the girls was told to instruct me in the ways of the bank and also docketing! I still don't know what that was all about; I'm not really into banks!

In the middle of January I realised that my period was late, not a sign of it, which was really unusual for me. I started

immediately thinking that I might be pregnant. I didn't tell

my husband, then. It got to February and my boobs were

getting sore and growing bigger and I missed my next

period. I knew that I was pregnant and I told my husband,

he was shocked. I started having morning sickness not just

in the mornings but also all through the day.

It was impossible for me to go to work and I had to hand

my notice in. They paid me for two more months. £100 in

all.

The doctor came to see me and felt my stomach and

confirmed the pregnancy. I felt really rough. My husband

was pleased about the pregnancy and so was his family.

My parents thought it was too soon.

They came up to Manchester to see us and were appalled

at the bed-sit and told my husband he must find a small

flat with more than one room especially now I was

expecting a baby. To give him his due he did just that and

we ended up in a flat on the top floor of a large Victorian house in Didsbury. It had a kitchen, a lounge, a bedroom and a bathroom; it was much better than the bed-sit. Now I was at home all day on my own I became bored again and depressed. My husband brought home a little black kitten for me, which I called Susie. I loved her. The morning, all day sickness continued and I found it hard to just do the washing up. My husband would come home to a mess and no supper. I think he must have been very patient with me and we never argued. Susie would claw her way up the eiderdown and snuggle next to us at night.

Around this time my husband was offered a job with a tyre company in Blackburn. The Job came with a flat above the shop and office, which meant that I would be close to him and not so much on my own. He took it and was expected to turn the business in that branch around to a profit. It had been making a loss. No pressure then! He had one other guy working with him called Walter.

Business was slow, mainly because the competition was hot. There were at least four other tyre companies along that long stretch of road. My husband worked hard to bring it round.

The flat was very nice and furnished in a modern style. There were two bedrooms, the lounge, then the hallway and bathroom and then the large kitchen and at the other end of the hallway a really big room. We used it as our bedroom for a while.

Meanwhile my pregnancy was progressing and I was monitored by the local GP practice.

I started to become anaemic and my blood was tested often. Eventually I was put on iron tablets and then it got so bad that I had to have iron injections in my, you guessed it, derriere! My behind looked very strange with stretch marks and brown stains. I felt exhausted most of the time. When I was seven months pregnant we travelled to Bristol to attend my older sister's wedding. She and her husband to be had been at university in Bristol where they met. The wedding was at a registry office; she looked lovely, very summery and hippy. I looked very pregnant in the photos. I missed my normally slight body.

We returned to Blackburn and started the countdown to the end of September. I had been given the 26th September as a possible day for the birth. The iron injections continued and they tried to get me to take folic acid, but it just made me throw up. The weather was hot and humid. On the 13th September 1970 I started getting excruciating pains down the left side of my stomach. My in laws were visiting that day. I went to bed and a doctor was called. It was a Sunday. He examined me and diagnosed a kidney infection. He had some antibiotics with him and gave me enough to last until the next day plus a prescription. He was concerned because I was so near to the end of the pregnancy but reassured my husband that I was not having labour pains.

The in-laws left, thank god and I took the medication. The pain lessened and I recovered during the next few days. By the end of that week I suddenly became very energetic and started doing all sorts of things like tidying up all my papers and the flat. On the Saturday I was manic and then about lunchtime I started having mild contractions. By teatime they were stronger and we still had to go into the town centre to buy me a dressing gown! All that evening the contractions continued but they were mild. We went to bed about ten and went off to sleep. At one in the morning I woke up suddenly in the middle of a very painful contraction. I woke my husband up and told him I thought the baby was coming. He panicked and phoned the maternity home. They told him to bring me in. Meanwhile I went to the loo and my waters broke while I was sitting there. After that the packed suitcase was grabbed and we got into my car, a grey Ford Anglia given to me by my Mother. It had four gears, three going forward and reverse. The MGA had been sold, as I was too large to get behind the wheel!

The Maternity home was called Bull Hill Maternity Home and was in Darwen a few miles down the road. The contractions came fast and furious and I wondered if the baby was going to arrive in the car. We arrived at about 1.45 am and went into the building.

I was put in a bed in a labour ward, which had three beds in it. At this point my husband left me. In those days husbands were not encouraged to hang around. I felt very alone and scared. I had no family nearby that would help me through all of this. I was examined and told that I was only about one centimetre dilated and that it would be ages.

Then I was given an enema but the tube wouldn't stay in

my back passage. It was a horrible experience. I ended up in the toilet after that and sat there for a good half hour as the world fell out of me. After that I was told to have a warm bath. I lay in that bath and looked at my stomach as it contracted and then relaxed, the pain was getting worse. I was then put back in bed and given an injection of pethidine. This put me to sleep and every so often I would jerk awake and cry out, as an agonising pain would cut like a knife low down in my groin at the front.

At about three in the morning an Indian lady was brought in and put in another bed. She lay there moaning as her labour progressed. As dawn broke about six o clock she was taken away to the delivery room, it was her third child I was told later. Meanwhile the agonising pains had stopped and I felt my body going into the transition stage between the first stage and the final stage, being, giving birth. I told the nurse that things had changed and she went and got the Sister who came and examined me and said, "this baby's coming", they got me out of bed and made me walk down the corridor to the delivery room! I thought the baby was going to drop out of me. I had two nurses, one on either side of me holding me up. In the delivery room they got me onto the table and I lay back, there was a large clock on the wall opposite me saying 7 am with the date showing 20th September 1970. I was given an injection and told to push when I felt like it and then pant, which I did without thinking. There was no pain in all of this and I just let my body take over. At 7.20 am my beautiful Son was born into this world. He cried, the cord was cut and he was wrapped up and given to me as I lay spent on the table.

I looked down at his face and he cried at me, the shock of coming out of his nice warm place inside me out into the bright light of the early morning written all over his little face.

I loved him.

After a while they took him away and put him in a cradle to the side of me where I could hear him gurgling to himself. I was given another injection to help the placenta to come out intact, which it did and I was told that although there was a tiny tear I wouldn't need any stitches in my nether regions.

I didn't care, I had got through all the worst and come out with a lovely baby son. They brought me a 'pot' of tea, literally, and I drank out of the special spout. It was wonderful! My husband on the other hand slept through the whole thing and didn't phone to see how I was until 10 that morning. He went down in my estimation at that point and never came back up.

11

The next fifteen months were the best in the whole of our marriage. We both loved our son and settled into a family life. Little Susie our cat had got herself pregnant while we were visiting our families one weekend and we returned to find her washing herself and about four tom cats lined up on the wall ! She eventually had four kittens, two black males and two black and amber females. They were gorgeous. We gave three away and kept one which we called Sam. I would have kept all of them if I could.

The months passed and I struggled with post-natal depression, my hormones were very imbalanced although at that time that sort of thing wasn't addressed properly by doctors and you were expected to just get on with it, it was part and parcel of being a woman they thought and said. Sometimes I just couldn't get up in the mornings. People would come into the tyre depot and ask how I was doing and my husband would say I was OK. I know that they thought it was odd that I didn't make an appearance with our son, but I just wasn't myself at all. The thing that interfered with my mental state and had been with me since I was eight was still with me and worse. I was still blocked off on quite a few levels mentally and struggled with meeting new people. My husband knew that I wasn't quite right when he married me and I know that he had severe doubts about going through with the marriage because of this although he never talked about it and even came to see me the night before the marriage to try and back out of it. Unfortunately, he met up with resistance in the form of my Father at the front door and was dispatched firmly. My Father had spent a good deal of money on the wedding and was not going to have it ruined because of an attack of pre-wedding nerves on the part of the groom. It was more than pre-wedding nerves and my Father knew this and so on some level did I.

My husband had taken on a lot marrying me and although

he was fond of me didn't have the love he should have had for me and neither me for him.

About fifteen months after the birth of our son, my husband came home one afternoon after a board meeting. He was not in a good mood and was distracted, I really struggled with him to tell me what had gone on. The upshot was that he had been given a months notice to leave the job. He said that he had resigned. Whether he had or whether they sacked him I don' t know.

So, he had no job and our accommodation was gone. He had no answers.
I phoned my parents that evening and told them what was going on. They both reassured me and said that there would be a home for us with them. I told my husband this. He seemed Ok with it because in truth we didn't have a choice.

12

We arrived back in Kettering with the little that we had and tried to settle in living with my parents and my younger sister. My parents were very good and had had the attic rooms made ready including a small kitchen made in one of the rooms. Fortunately there were two bathrooms in the main house. We lived on the 'dole' as it was called then while my husband looked for work. I was offered a job at the local private school where I had been a pupil, teaching Piano, I worked two mornings per week. It was hard for me because of my brain and mind problem but I was determined and I had to keep it well hidden if I was to keep the job. My husband decided that he would go on a government training scheme to learn to be a TV engineer, this meant that he would be training away from home in

Worksop each week and would come home at weekends. My Mother in law was worried that it would drive us apart and in the end she was right, it did.

I struggled while he was away, with my health and looking after our Son and working at the school. I also took on pupils to teach at home and used my parents piano and the study to teach in. I joined a local Drama Society which I loved and acted in quite a few plays with them. The director was a lovely Indian man who also wrote his own plays one of which was called 'Nirvana' which we performed in the British Drama Guild competition. I think we came first in our region.

My husband came home at weekends and didn't like the fact that I was trying to get on with my life and having outside interests. I think he thought that I should cleave to him and our son and that was it. At this point after a particularly bad row I went downstairs in the late evening to get a drink and my Dad followed me down. We sat in the study and talked and I told him that I just couldn't stay in the marriage, he was very good and listened but I knew it would be up to me in the end.

My husband's course ended and he got a job locally in the town. This was before Christmas in 1974. Around Christmas time I felt something physical 'give' in my brain but I didn't tell anyone. I was already on medication.

In the new year, February 1975 I went on the contraceptive pill. We had moved into our own house which was old and needed a lot of work doing on it. My husband had chosen it because it was a double plot and he wanted the space so that he would have room for his beloved old cars. He did not think about the needs of a young wife and child and there was only an outside toilet and an old bath in the existing kitchen. My older sister and her first husband came and helped us decorate. Meanwhile my husband and I just weren't getting on at all and I could feel the marriage slipping away. The contraceptive pill meanwhile was playing havoc with my mind and body and I sank into the black hole of a major depression and my emotional outbursts became worse. I knew that I wasn't right but just didn't think of the contraceptive pill as the reason I just thought it was the state of my marriage. I persuaded my husband to take a day off to try and talk about our problems, actually I screamed at him and told him that it was over if he wouldn't.

So he did. We took our son and drove to Norfolk to get right away from it all. We talked normally for the first time in months over a meal and drink in a pub. We drove back slowly in the evening through the Norfolk countryside. The evening was wet and cold. As we drove down a particularly narrow country road I started to feel really odd in my mind as if I had been there before. At the end of the road there were two big gates obviously leading to a country house, I just felt as though I should be going through those gates to get home. I said nothing to my husband about the strangeness of it and we drove on. By the time we reached Cambridge I felt really ill in my mind and made him stop the car. At that time there was a man on the loose called 'the Cambridge ripper' who had been attacking women. In my distorted mind I thought my husband was this person and made him drive to a pub near the A1. I called the police from the pub, I was really frightened, so was my husband and took our son and left me there on my own. When the police came I was in tears about it all and said I didn't feel well. The police were very good, saw what was happening to me and phoned my parents. My Dad and my younger sister came to get me. They were both very stressed and angry with me, which made me worse. They took me to my parents house where my Mum was waiting, by this time my mind had gone completely and I told them I needed a Doctor. Nobody listened to me and I was marginalized. My Mum told me to go to bed and they would get the doctor in the morning. I waited until they were going to bed and saw my dad lock the front door, I thought he was locking me in. Because of this I crept down the stairs, went to the kitchen and got a small kitchen knife for protection and proceeded to climb out of the front lounge window. I ran down the road, stopped two young people and told them I needed the police. I ran on and started up another road where I knocked on a front door and scared the living daylights out of two elderly women asking them to get the police.

I left them and continued to run and knocked on another door. The gentleman talked to me through the letter box and phoned the police. I crouched in the front garden behind a tree with the knife in front of me. The police came and I showed myself, I gave them the knife and they got me in the police car. They asked for my name which I gave as 'Anna Hamilton' and I asked for' Richard'. I had completely lost all sense of reality and had seemed to slip into another place and time. They took me to the local police station where I was examined for other weapons by a female police officer. They called my parents who were going mad with worry as they had found that I had left the house through the window. Again my Father came for me and I screamed at him that he was not my father. Eventually I calmed down enough for my dad to get me in the car and he asked me where I would like to go, to my husband and son or back with him, nowhere seemed right but I chose my husband and son. That night I lay in bed next to my husband and stared at the ceiling where a large eye stared back at me.

The next morning a police woman stood outside the front

door, a social worker arrived and a psychiatrist came to speak to me. My Mum and Dad were in the next room. My Husband sat next to me on the sofa while Minnie Ripperton sang 'loving you' over and over in my mind. The psychiatrist, one Dr Took, was very nice and Scottish. He talked to my husband about what had happened and my husband said that I should be 'put away' to which the psychiatrist replied that it was up to me and that I would make a choice. For the first time in my life I felt as though I was being listened to.

I was given the choice of going to St Crispins Hospital to have a rest because I hadn't slept for 48 hours or to stay at home and sleep over the weekend and then attend the Mayfair day hospital on the Monday as a day patient. Both were Mental hospitals. I chose the latter. I slept all the weekend helped by drugs that the psychiatrist had left for me and given to me by my husband. On the Monday morning I entered the next phase of my life as

<u>'a mental patient'</u>

_Part 2

Mentality (with physicality thrown in for good measure)

13

The Mayfair Day Hospital was in a house that I used to

play with my friend ' Mima' when I was young and also

where she had lived and I was very disconcerted to find

myself back in that house as a mentally ill patient. I

couldn't get my head around the dichotomy of the two times

I had been there. Also my parents house was at the back

of the 'Mayfair'. It all felt so strange to me and muddle-y. I

felt rested and positive that they would help me. I was

introduced to the psychologist that would be on my case.

He was older than me and had a beard, his eyes were the

same colour as mine and I found that significant. He asked

me to fill in a questionnaire which took me about an hour and being my totally honest and straightforward self I filled it in with all the details as I saw it. The result was that I was put on Largactil a rather nasty chemical anti-psychotic drug. I was put on 150 mg per day, a large dose. My skin became hyper sensitive to the sun and I had to sit in the shade. They talked about me having had a psychotic break. I was drugged up and dopey and couldn't keep my eyes open in the therapy meetings we had to take part in. There was always a meeting in the mornings where the patients , psychiatrist , psychologist and nurses would sit together in a circle in silence until someone could bear it no longer and start to speak. I didn't understand the purpose of it and hardly said a word, I felt as though I was in an alien world with an alien race of beings that didn't speak my language. Every so often, the husband of one of the patients would arrive and shout and get violent towards her while we were in these meetings. He was always removed but it was shocking to see him in action and I felt for his wife.

Meanwhile the psychologist had taken a fancy to me and started to pursue me. My marriage was on the rocks, my mind was ill and I was vaguely flattered that I should be pursued. I thought it was innocent until after I slept with him in his filthy council flat and was seeing an image of 'Kali, the Indian death goddess' on the wall, I quickly took some medication and got out of there. He treated me very badly from then on saying that he was seeing someone else and even bringing her to my front door one day. He stood me up several times and I should have trusted my instincts to stay away from him. It was difficult because he was professionally involved with me and shouldn't have been cavorting with a patient. He tried to explain it away to his superior, the psychiatrist, Dr Took by coming 'clean' as he put it. I was very vulnerable because of the state of my mind and unused to playing the game of relationships at that time and was taken advantage of. He was in my life for 3 years, he stuck like glue, eventually I got rid of him as he moved away. About six years later, out of the blue, I had a phone call from him and he told me he had been 'struck off' and was unable to carry on his work as a psychologist as it had been found that he had a history of coming on sexually to his young female patients wherever he had worked. What bad luck for me that I was caught up in his web of lust and deceit at a time when I needed love and care.

My marriage ended after more arguments with my husband and when I found him with another woman. One night when he came in at 3 am he screamed at me for about an hour and told me I had made my bed and I must lie in it. I would say it takes two to make a bad marriage and he played his deceitful part in it by marrying me in the first place while there was doubt in his mind. My heart was elsewhere and that was what led to my mental breakdown in the first place. But nobody asked me and I kept it to myself and still do mostly! My heart was with my first love who proposed marriage at the age of eight with a lovely gold and sparkly ring and getting down on one knee to ask me. I felt fear because of my strange mental state at the time but I will always love him even though he shunned me because of his lack of understanding of my mental problems and the advice his parents gave him about my illnesses. I cannot settle with another because they are not 'right'.

I would rather die being true to my feelings than try to be with another and that is how it will be in this this life unless he comes to me which I think he has tried to do, but put off by the sight of another man at my front door who has proved to be yet another frog!

Please try again when the time is right in this life or the next……….

14

My life continued. In the end I pretended that I was OK mentally even though I felt deathly depressed and got out of the mental day hospital after 9 months of being there. I lived on benefits and agreed with my husband that our son and I should continue to live in the marital home. My Mum had paid for improvements to the house and we had an indoor bathroom and toilet and a bigger kitchen/diner. I tried to settle in there but we were not there long as my husband arrived on the doorstep one Sunday and our son let him in and he said he was coming back. I later learned that his motive was purely money, no love involved. My son and I had to leave the house and we were effectively on the streets. My Mum and Dad took my son in and I was farmed out to stay in my parents friends houses. I would have lost my benefits if I had stayed at my parents house. My Mother was so angry that day that she got me in the car and we drove round the town looking for a little house to buy for me and my son. We found one and I still live in it to this day, my Mum used some of her inheritance from her Father to buy it. I managed to pay most of it back over the years. It is my sanctuary. Determined that I would do what I should have done when I was 18, I applied to go to university, a mature student, to become a teacher in music and drama.

I was accepted into University but ended up studying Music and Dance as the main drama day coincided with the main music day. How absurd to put two main arts subjects on the same day. I enjoyed dancing but found the anatomy and physiology difficult to learn. The three years at university have been some of the best in my life. I loved singing and playing the piano and dancing, I felt in my element. I felt stimulated mentally and physically. I took the lead role of 'Yum Yum' in The Mikado by Gilbert and Sullivan and also 'Mabel' in The Pirates of Penzance. I wrote piano music for a fellow student called John to dance to and we performed it in front of a large audience, me on piano and him dancing. I also choreographed and danced my own solo at the end of term and college dance performance and had a standing ovation. I sang a duet from Britten's 'Ceremony of Carols' in a large church.

Towards the end of my time at University I went for an interview for a job which unknown to me covered a 'sink' council estate in its catchment area. We were told to take any job we were offered as jobs were at a premium by the University. There were only two candidates for this particular job as a music teacher. My competitor was a younger student and they offered her the job first but she turned it down.

Consequently the job was offered to me and I took it. The University was very pleased as I was the first student teacher to get a job.

The last term came to an end and I had passed the course pretty well including a 'credit ' in Music.

During the school holidays I went in to the new school to help the Head of Music get things ready for the next term.

Even then I had my doubts as to whether I would be able to do justice to my work as a teacher as I was a creative teacher and as time went by I realised that this school was run not as a comprehensive as it should have been but almost as a grammar school where everyone was put into streams A B and C and then remedial. The headmaster was awful and had one eye that looked away from you when he was talking to you which was very disconcerting as you didn't know which eye to look at.

The deputy head looked like a male gorilla (no insult to gorilla's intended) even though she was female!

I knew within two weeks of teaching there that I just didn't want to be at that school. I was oppressed by the system. One example was an English lesson and I was teaching my own class about a William Shakespeare play and we moved the desks back so that they could 'act' it out. They loved doing this and we all were having a good lesson. In the middle of this the door was flung open by the headmaster and he shouted to my class to put the desks back and for several of my students to go to his study. He completely usurped my position as teacher and didn't even say anything to me. The rest of my class just looked at me not understanding what had happened. To be honest I didn't know either. I did know that I didn't want to be there. Another odd thing happened, I passed my English teaching really well but failed my Music teaching. I was told that I would be assessed by the music inspector teaching an 'A' band lesson. In fact he barged in to a remedial class that I was teaching. We were listening to 'Peter and the Wolf' and they were drawing pictures to go with the story. They were fine and settled but when he came in they started swearing and asking what the f...k was this man doing in the lesson. Most of these children were West Indian and from the 'sink' estate and could hardly read but they were well versed in swear vocabulary.

I knew that this had not gone down well and I was terrified about teaching in front of him after the morning break. The lesson was ok but I had lost my confidence. He failed me, I was mortified, I had spent three years training to teach Music and had had no training in teaching English and yet passed the second and failed the first. It was bizarre. I took it to the NUT, National Union of Teachers, who took on my case. I was given a full apology from the County Inspectorate and told that it would have been different in another school. They left it open for me if I wanted to go back into the state system.

All this had taken its toll on my health and I had to take time off, in fact I never went back there. I was paid until the September and then I was on my own financially with my son to bring up without any help from his father except a small maintenance payment of £56.00 per month.

Meanwhile my son had been at boarding school as he had won a scholarship as a Chorister at Canterbury Cathedral the year before! How proud I was of him.

I did cleaning work and I was offered a job at a Public School teaching Piano. I took the job at the school and also started teaching from home nearly every evening during the week.

I continued working in this way for 14 years but found it difficult to make ends meet and struggled with everything including my health and money. The 'thing' affecting my brain was still ever present and I was taking Melleril an anti- psychotic for my supposed mental illness.

My next experience, which nearly killed me, was having my four wisdom teeth out at Kettering General Hospital. I was 30 at the time.

I had visited the dentist, for a check up and he took an X-ray of my whole jaw and told me my wisdom teeth would have to come out, as there was no room for them.

I was referred to the hospital. I went and met the specialist who would be removing said teeth under general anaesthetic. He was very scathing about my teeth in general and asked why my dentist had not dealt with the caries in my wisdom teeth!

I was booked in and went for the pre-op appointment, which was carried out by a very young and inexperienced oriental female doctor. I told her about the anti psychotic medication I was on and trusted that this would be taken into consideration. This particular medication called 'Melleril' (thioridazine) had a side effect of lowering an enzyme in the body called Cholinesterase. I was unaware of this and when it came time for the operation I went nearly to my demise without knowing it. I was given a drug called Scoline, which relaxes all the muscles of the body including the breathing muscles round the lungs so that the anaesthetist can take over the breathing for the body. The drug interacts with the enzyme cholinesterase in the body which keeps the body breathing on it's own. Because of the level of cholinesterase being very low in my body due to the action of the anti psychotic drug 'Melleril', when it came to bringing me 'back' after the operation I was unable to breathe for myself, apparently there was a huge panic and I was put on a ventilator to keep me alive until my body recovered from the action of the drug Scoline. It is now recognised that a bad reaction to Scoline can cause an Apnoea. Somewhere along the line the surgeon had not done his homework on the anti psychotic effect on the cholinesterase in my body, or the Anaesthetist didn't look or the oriental doctor had forgotten to put it in my file.

When I came round eventually the nurse attending me said' we're glad to have you back Anne'. I asked what had happened and was told sketchily of the events.

I was appalled and when the Specialist came to see me he looked frightened and kept his distance from the bed. If I had been in my right mind I would have pursued with a complaint but couldn't seem to get any clear details of what had happened from any of the staff. Just another frightening medical event!

When I was 34 I started to bleed in between periods. I was referred to the hospital where they proceeded to examine me internally and told me I had a polyp attached to my cervix. They removed it and that cleared up.

Then I started to bleed heavily each month (more than usual) when having my period. I was referred to the hospital again for a D&C. Basically they scrape out the rubbish inside your uterus. They did this, but I had a bad reaction to the anaesthetic and had a crushing headache afterwards. Normally it was a day procedure but they kept me in overnight and then forgot about me, as I was the only one left in the ward. It wasn't until the cleaner came and saw me in the bed the next morning that it was realised that I was there. They did apologise and brought me breakfast but obviously there had been a breakdown in communication somewhere. Good job I was still alive!

At the age of 36 I became very ill with very heavy periods again and was haemorrhaging every month. It became very distressing and I was becoming very anaemic. I 'flooded' at a visit to the doctors surgery in the waiting room. As I got up to go into the doctor's room, the blood ran down the inside of my legs and there were huge red clots. I ran into his room and he saw what was happening, to say that he panicked is an understatement! He eventually managed to get the receptionist up the stairs and she took me into a medical room downstairs where she left me to deal with all the blood and clots. Eventually he came downstairs to see me and I asked him what was I going to do about it. He told me that I would have to have a hysterectomy. (At least he had seen it all in Technicolor action and I didn't have to prove it to him! He was one of those who needed a lot of convincing!)

I felt that I might have had a miscarriage as I had missed my period the month before and was entangled in yet another unfortunate relationship.

I went privately to see a gynaecologist. I was examined and he told me I had big fibroids in my uterus and because I was haemorrhaging every month a hysterectomy was the thing to do.

The last period I had was a humdinger and I called my GP in as I felt as though I was departing this life. The blood test he took showed that I was running on about half the red blood cells that I should have had and I was put on a large dose of Iron tablets. Fortunately I was booked in for the hysterectomy 4 weeks after that at the beginning of December 1987.

On December 2nd I was admitted to Kettering General

Hospital to a private room and I had to have a blood transfusion, 4 pints in all, 3 ordinary and 1 plasma. It took 14 hours for it to all go in to my body. The next day I wandered around feeling shell shocked as my body assimilated the new blood.

On December 4th 1987 I was wheeled down to the operating theatre and watched the ceiling lights go by above me. I felt nauseous and my next period had started to show itself. I was glad to go to sleep under the anaesthetic and leave this world behind for a while.

Afterwards when I woke up my Mother and Son were by my side, I was very groggy and swam in and out of consciousness. It took me 24 hours to come out of the anaesthetic properly. The pain was being controlled by Morphine through a drip and when the anaesthetist came to see me he told me I was on Heroin at that time. The Surgeon came to see me and told me that the largest fibroid was the size of an orange and there were other smaller ones, they had been sent to the Path Lab to see if they were cancerous or infected with TB. Fortunately for me they were not so I breathed a huge sigh of relief. So did everyone else!

I remained in hospital for 10 days and then was allowed to go to my Parents home. They were both in their 70's then so it was a lot for them to cope with. I was weak for at least a month and then slowly started to get some strength back. My mental health remained the same as it had since I was 8 – bad. Eventually I came home and tried to rest. After another 2 months I had to return to work and realised I had gone back too soon but had to carry on as I needed the money to survive.

After all that I had another respite apart from the ever present mental problem which pervaded my entire life. I managed to carry on working at the School and at home but I had to borrow on the equity of the house to cover myself when I was too ill to work.

I stayed at the School until I was unceremoniously made redundant. Just a terse letter, no notice was given, at the end of the Summer Term in 1994 saying there would be no work for me in September. A new Head of Music had taken over and obviously this was his 'new' way ! I had to fight through the Citizen's Advice Bureau to get some redundancy pay and eventually the School settled out of court, no publicity wanted of course.

I managed to build up my work over the next 6 years until at one point I had 60 students altogether per week. My money worries were at bay for a while. In December 2000 I visited my GP about my painful right knee, he said I had 'crepitus', a crackling as it moved but did not offer to move forward with it by sending me to a specialist, I sighed, resigned to more bullshit. At the same appointment he informed me that I would have to come off Melleril (thioridazine) as there had been a Government Directive that all patients should come off it as it had been found to be detrimental to the heart. He told me that my heart could just stop. I was very shocked at this bit of news as I had been on it for about 24 years and wondered how I was going to manage to get off it in the 5 weeks he advised as it was very addictive. I told my family that I had to come off it, at this point in time I was not given or advised to have a suitable substitute although 'Sandoz' the Pharmaceutical company and manufacturer had advised that a suitable substitute should be given, I found this out later. As the weeks went on with my heavy workload continuing and as I cut the drug as gradually as I could I felt my mental state altering. By February 2001 I was beginning to feel very unwell and asked for a home visit from my GP, one Dr Wildgoose. He came and he and I sat in my back room and discussed how I was feeling. I asked to be referred to the Mental Health Team for some help with coming off the drug. He refused my request saying that they were 'too busy'!!! I asked for something to help me and he left me with a prescription for 'Promazine'. I took the promazine that evening and within a hour I was having painful burning sensations all round my midriff in the nerve endings. I realised I was having an adverse reaction to the drug and called my Son who came and also my younger Sister. I ended up on the toilet with severe diarrhoea and was shaking badly. My son phoned 'Keydoc' and was advised by a Doctor that I was having an allergic reaction and that it would take at least eight hours to start to leave my system. My Son stayed over for the night even though he had just moved in to a different house that day with his partner and she was forced by circumstance to spend that first night alone in the new home. The next day I phoned my GP and told him what had happened, he advised me not to take it again but did not give me anything else to help with the withdrawal of the Melleril.

So, I continued and came off Melleril completely by the beginning of March. I continued to work but by the middle of March I was beginning to be psychotic, a backlash of coming off the drug. I was finding it hard to concentrate when I was teaching and my dreams were vivid and frightening. I had friends and family round on my birthday, the 24th and was very manic. At the end of March I had to stop teaching due to exhaustion and the psychosis. In the first week of April I spoke to my Mother on the phone and told her I was very ill. Both my parents came round and my Mother told my Father to go and get a Doctor from the surgery. Fortunately for me it was a female competent one and after talking to me she got a Psychiatrist and a community psychiatric nurse to come and see me straight away. I explained what had happened and the psychiatrist told me I was suffering from Bi-polar disorder and drug

withdrawal and put me on Olanzapine (anti psychotic),

Librium (tranquillizer) and Zopiclone (sleeping pill). A week

later he also put me on Citalopram

(Anti-depressant). I spent a week in bed mostly asleep.

The female doctor was appalled at the way I had just been

left by my GP and I remember him coming in to visit me

and attempting to 'fluff' his way out of his appalling neglect.

He had led me on a 'wild goose' chase for years. I did

report him in letter form to the Practise Manager but it was

all passed back to him and he sent me a letter repudiating

my concerns. Blatant lies, by him. I also sent a letter to

the Government Health Ombudsman dealing with these

matters but was told to go down a level and report it to

another body of people, (round and round).

Meanwhile I was unable to work and lost about half my students, so my income was slashed once again. I had to cash in my pension early and lost about £2000 in the process to keep myself going financially until my private sickness insurance kicked in and some state benefits. This meant that I would have no private pension when I was 65. It took me a long time to recover from all that and I have never been able to build up my students to that extent since then.

Meanwhile, my knee had got worse and in 2002 I went into hospital to have an 'arthroscopy'. The Surgeon said that the cartilage was very damaged. He repaired it as best he as could and I tried to recover. I limped and hobbled everywhere. When I returned to see him he said I would be best to have a knee replacement. The thought of having metal and plastic inside my body made me feel ill. About four days before the date of the operation which had been arranged, I phoned the surgeon's secretary and cancelled it, I was very fearful now about anything to do with medical procedures.

In 2009 I was booked in at Kettering General Hospital to have a Knee replacement, it still didn't feel right but the pain was so great that I felt there was no other choice at that time. The night before I was in tears and prayed to the higher to look after me and if it was not meant to be then to present a way out. On the morning of the operation my Son took me up to the hospital at 7.00am.I hobbled my way up to the ward I was booked into and the proceedings started. I was shown to my bed and the anaesthetist arrived to examine me, my surgeon was nowhere to be seen. There was another Surgeon talking to another patient and he was giving me quick looks every so often. My Son left me and as I started to unpack my belongings a young Indian Doctor came rushing down the corridor, in his hand a green folder, he skidded to a stop outside the ward doors and looked around, he saw me and asked if I was Miss Scott.' Yes' I said and he proceeded to inform me that the special part for my knee had not been ordered and that the operation would not go forward. It turned out that the waiting list office had neglected to look at my file to see if I needed anything out of the ordinary and had put me on an earlier date as they had a space. My Surgeon was away on holiday at that time as well and when I made a formal complaint to the hospital trust I had a letter of apology from him. It was not his fault it was lack of checking work by the waiting list office. Just another incident!!! Or another helping hand from the higher to save me from neglect.

Meanwhile my neighbour across the road had introduced me to 'Reiki', an alternative healing method, she offered to train me in the art for nothing as she needed to practise

herself as she had only just become a Reiki Master. During

this time my spirituality was growing and I had reorganised

my house and created a 'healing room' upstairs. I also

redecorated downstairs and had a very ugly fireplace taken

out in my front room. I settled down a bit more and began

to study alternative healing methods such as Colour

Therapy, Herbs and the use of Astrology charts to

determine a person's health or lack of it, also flower

remedies and tissue salts. For years,30 odd, I had been

studying the ancient arts of Astrology, tarot reading, the I

Ching and The Tao, now I was trying to link it all together

when finding out about my health, with some success. I

had bought many books over the years on health trying to

find out what had caused my difficult mental state when I

was so young and I had at this time come to the conclusion

that it had had something to do with my onset of puberty

and trouble in my endocrine system. I pursued this line of

thought and read about how too much oestrogen could cause severe psychosis.

In 2010 during a visit to a psychiatrist for a routine check up, as I was still under the mental health team after coming off Melleril (thioridazine), my views on this were confirmed by a locum standing in for my usual Doctor. I gave him a very short history of my illness and he agreed that it would indeed be possible that my illness could be caused by too much oestrogen although this had not been considered or followed up by anyone over the years….WHY? I walked out of the building that day and felt that a bright white light had been switched on in my mind having had my own diagnosis possibly confirmed. After all these years,56 to be precise, of being locked away from the world, trapped in a grey, distorted colourless reality, maybe at last I was getting near to the cause.

Meanwhile my life continued and I was able to do further research. I was also able to do some teaching although I was suffering from 'burn out' after 40 years of doing this while coping with the mental side of things. I started using a crystal pendulum and bought myself a book of pendulum Charts. I had had the quartz pendulum for about ten years and had kept it safe in a velvet bag, now I took it out of the bag and started to acquaint myself with it and tried using the charts to start to find out about 'things'!!!!

One of things I was able to find out was other peoples motivations for their particular actions either towards me or other people which proved to be most enlightening. This was especially so regarding behaviour and actions from all the Doctors I had seen over the years and has helped me to come to terms with my experiences in the NHS. 'Physician heal thyself' and 'The truth will set you free' had become very real tenets of faith for me over the years, although I had been born into a Christian family and taken to church every Sunday while growing up unfortunately there was and has been a distinct lack of understanding regarding my health situation by family members and others who should have known better, apart from my Mother and Son who have been my 'Rocks'. The Spiritual 'Higher' has sent many 'helpers' over the years all of which have helped me to stay on my 'path' of finding a way through the maze of ill health and spiritual discovery.

My work on the Pendulum Charts revealed to me that I had a small benign growth in my right ovary and that it had been there for most of my life. Consequently when I approached the age of puberty and my endocrine system started clicking in, my right ovary was not functioning correctly and disturbed my whole endocrine system including my Pituitary gland and hypothalamus in my brain which guide the functioning of the system, thus my strange

and difficult mental state for all these years, cut off and

living in a mental prison. There are many prisons of

differing types but the prison of being locked in a body that

is not functioning as it should and a mind that is very

limited and dull because of it, is one of the worst in my

experience. I am sure that all the people that have similar

conditions suffer in the same way, that of being totally

aware but unable to communicate and express that

awareness and also having to deal with the ignorance and

stigma that comes with it. My heart goes out to you all.

I had been studying the work on Colour therapy by

Dinshah, an expert who was put through a court case in

the US to prove his findings of the healing power of Colour

in the early 20th century, it was proved that it worked

although it was 'poo poohed' by the powers that were then

and still are. I arranged two lamps in my healing room to

start healing the growth in my ovary. I was to use the colour Orange for five weeks each day for eighteen minutes per treatment every day without fail. The colour had to be shined on bare skin, so one lamp directed to my Solar plexus which radiates to all the energy centre's (chakras) within the body and another directed to the soles of my feet, also a direct line to all the other chakras.

I started this at the beginning of this year, 2015 in January and managed to discipline myself to carry out the treatment every day. After five weeks I had started to feel somewhat better physically and my mental state was improving slowly. As of now, the middle of May 2015,at last I feel as though I am gradually getting free of my very difficult journey through the quagmire of my mental illness. The world is coming back into order for me although I still have a way to go with my poorly knees. I have started a healing program for my legs and knees that involves Colour healing, vitamins, EFA's (Omega oils 3,6,9) L - carnitine ,an amino acid, Tissue salts and flower remedies to help with emotional imbalances and it is working but the self discipline needed to carry it out is very intense. It is now July 2015 and I have had quite a few false starts with my most recent healing plan for my legs but I am determined to carry on with it.

Now I must bring my story to a close. I hope it will help all the people who have or are suffering with some sort of dis-ease of the body and mind and to know that there are alternative remedies that do work if you are prepared for them to take time, discipline and diligence. My most recent visit to the NHS involved a severe nose bleed which wouldn't stop in April 2015. I would like to say that I was treated with the utmost care apart from having to be trundled over in a very rickety ambulance to Northampton

General Hospital as Kettering had no Ear, Nose and Throat staff on duty at the weekend, another Government cut on our most needed services. I was kept there overnight and then trundled back with others in a very old ambulance bus that threw us around, hardly the most caring and comfortable service for sick and ill people but then why would a health service offer that?

The End.

Afterword

There are many caring and compassionate people that work in our overworked health system and I thank all the people down the line that actually gave me the time of day on a ratio of about 2:100. I bless you all, few as you were.

August 2015

I had a bad fall down my stairs on the 19th. No bones broken (a miracle) but quite a few contusions and a severe bang to the head. I was x-ray- ed and CT 'd and then sent home, I am recovering.

e.